# Senior Workouts

### Stay Fit and Healthy

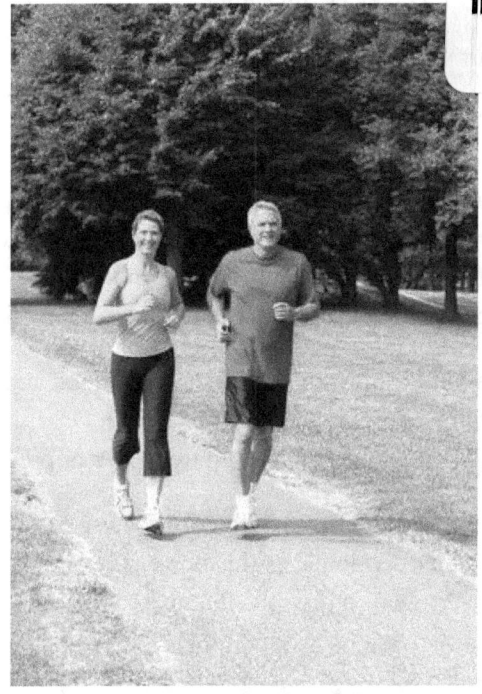

## Health Learning Series

### M. Usman

### Mendon Cottage Books

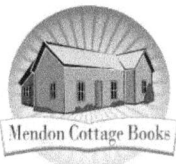

### *JD-Biz Publishing*

### Disclaimer

The information is this book is provided for informational purposes only. It is not intended to be used and medical advice or a substitute for proper medical treatment by a qualified health care provider. The information is believed to be accurate as presented based on research by the author.

The contents have not been evaluated by the U.S. Food and Drug Administration or any other Government or Health Organization and the contents in this book are not to be used to treat cure or prevent disease.

The author or publisher is not responsible for the use or safety of any diet, procedure or treatment mentioned in this book. The author or publisher is not responsible for errors or omissions that may exist.

### Warning

The Book is for informational purposes only and before taking on any diet, treatment or medical procedure, it is recommended to consult with your primary health care provider.

Our books are available at

1. Amazon.com
2. Barnes and Noble
3. Itunes
4. Kobo
5. Smashwords
6. Google Play Books

# Table of Contents

# Preface

Your body does not retain its original quality in terms of shape, strength, flexibility, etc. as you age. With the passage of time, the body loses its original properties and weakens; the heart pumps blood at a slower pace, the bones become more brittle, the veins become worn out and so on. In order to maintain the body in its healthy state, a planned physical routine is necessary. Just because you're aged 50 plus, doesn't mean the time to take care of your body has ended. On the contrary, the time has just come. It is very vital for senior individuals to take care of their body right from the start, to ensure longevity and a comfortable adult life. In a study by the Agency for Healthcare Research and Quality, it was found that over 85% of US Adults don't exercise in any regular way, which can cause an increase in the risk of serious cardiovascular, structural, and immune diseases. The book will provide comprehensive support to every adult citizen looking to rid himself of common yet irritating conditions caused by aging. The benefits are basically divided into two categories:

1.     Psychological

2.     Physical

Both will be explained up to great satisfaction in the book, after which the reader will be taken through a number of types of exercises through which he/she can benefit. All in all, your life is about to change, so get ready!

# Benefits of Exercise

## Chapter # 1: What good does it bring?

Exercise can induce a number of benefits on the human body irrespective of its age. Thus, stressing the advantages of a good workout is more than enough in boosting the morale of an elderly person to engage in physical activities. Exercise has countless benefits like protecting against chronic diseases, boosting immunity, improving cardiovascular organs, etc. along with cognitive ones which stretches a person's life. The complete list of benefits will be given at the end, but first a little explanation of the major benefits:

### 1.     Improved heart health:

In the US alone over 13.5 million individuals are diagnosed with heart disease, out of which, 1.5 million are sufferers of heart attacks. This risk of heart attacks increases with age and lack of physical activities, so just imagine what both these factors would do in conjunction. The primary reason for this elevated risk level is the weakening of the heart which can be fixed through proper exercise. Firstly, the exercise decreases the amount of LDL or bad cholesterol by increasing the amount of HDL or good cholesterol; this leads to unclogged arteries which is a big deciding factor in heart diseases. Secondly, it strengthens the heart which stabilizes the workload, because after all, the heart is just a muscle.

### 2.     Reduced Blood pressure:

One of the other major reasons as to why seniors adopt exercise is the reduction in high blood pressure. On its own, high blood pressure isn't a bad thing, but with the passage of time it can have life-altering effects and also with the passage of time, the blood pressure increases. It is approximated that almost 50 million people in the US alone have high blood pressure. Exercise can have a positive effect on a person's cardiovascular hygiene and can protect from all of the following high blood pressure risks:

- An increase in blood pressure means unhealthy blood vessels, which means major organ damage. What sounds really alarming is the fact that if the damage reaches the eye, it can result in blindness.

- High blood pressure increases the risk of stroke which is a condition where a clot forms in the brain, halting blood flow. The most obvious outcome is death if not treated immediately.

- As a result of high blood pressure, it is much easier for the plaque to build up on the walls of the arteries which means that eventually blood flow to the brain will be restricted leading to a decrease in cognitive skills.

- Reduced blood pressure means reduced fat levels which have a wide array of benefits alone. Exercise therefore reduces fat levels by reducing the blood pressure and also by natural physical activity.

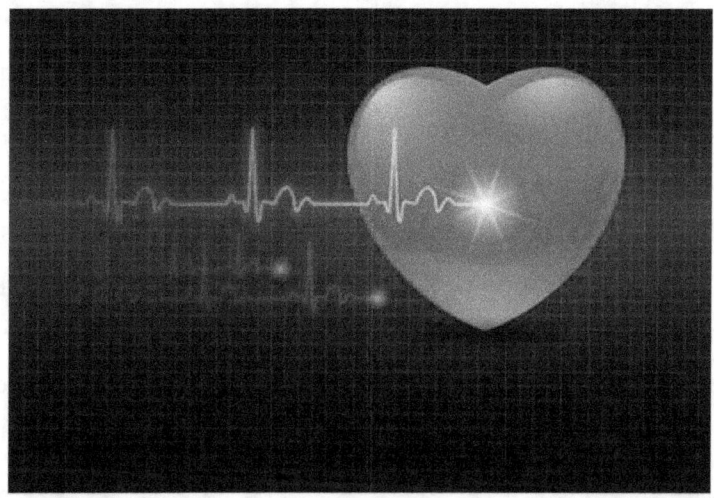

### 3. Better lungs:

An increase in physical activity means an automatic increase in oxygen demand; this means that one way or another the lungs will have to adapt to uptake a higher quantity of oxygen. This will induce an ideal benefit which will allow seniors to perform more tasks and become resilient in everyday life.

### 4. Bone and Muscle maintenance.

Regular exercise provides a great enterprise to bring back life into one's muscles and bones. Diseases like osteoporosis get worse with age and the only realistic way to stop them from affecting routine life is exercise. When bones are put under stress, they become stronger. For example when a person lifts weights, he/she puts stress on the bones and this makes them stronger, which is a plus for seniors. But, the physical activity shouldn't be too rigorous or else the senior will only end up injuring his/her own body. In addition to the bones, exercise would also strengthen the muscles which will naturally mean more power. Even though power is not really a requirement of a senior citizen, healthy muscles will ensure that the person is able to carry out daily chores easily, in case a supporting person is not available. All in all, exercise would prevent you from becoming a slouch by keeping the back and chest muscles in shape.

5.    **Reducing Fat levels:**

It is common knowledge that any physical activity increases body temperature which in turn reduces fat levels. High fat levels are linked with other conditions like heart disease or high blood pressure, so taking down fat levels can have expanded benefits. Furthermore, reduced fat levels mean that less pressure would now be put on joints and bones, which adds to a person's stamina and reduction in common arthritis problems.

6.    **Common cancers:**

There isn't rock hard evidence that links exercise to reduced cancer, but a few links have been found that imply a reduction in cancer risk through physical activity in the elderly. For women, exercise performed regularly can reduce the risk of uterine as well as breast cancers by reducing fat as well as estrogen levels. Estrogen is known to help in increasing cancer growth, so by normalizing estrogen levels, cancer risk is reduced. Exercise can also reduce the risk of prostate and colon cancer. You might already know that colon cancer is the top cancer in men who are aged above 50. Researchers are finding out that exercise can move food through the large intestine with a faster pace which reduces the time waste is stored in the colon; this in turn leads to reduced cancer risk.

7.    **Better Immunity:**

With the passage of time, seniors lose their immunity. They get sick more often and fail to show the same strength in the face of common diseases they could decades ago. Exercise has shown to have a positive effect on immunity according to a Dutch study. The study was conducted on 117 individuals, men and women, who were aged at 79 on average. The results showed that increased physical activity boosted immunity and hardened resistance against diseases.

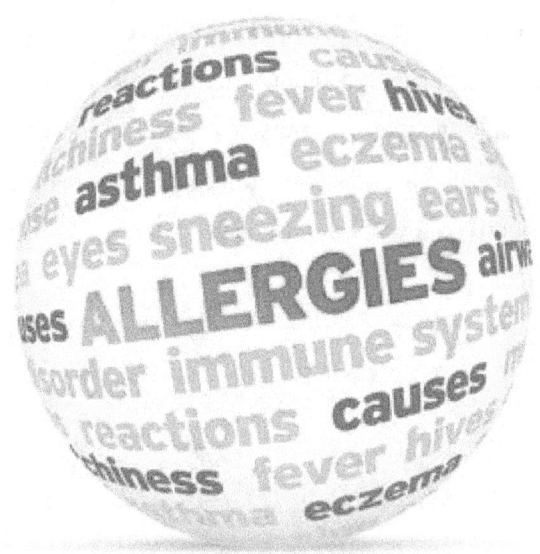

## 8.    Psychological Benefits:

Most people think of exercise as an entity which helps the body physically, but realistically speaking, exercise also has a number of psychological benefits. For starters, it makes a person feel good. It boosts a person's self-confidence and esteem which really helps a person perform better in day-to-day tasks. The scientific reason behind this good-feeling is the release of endorphins, which is a hormone that induces calm and serenity. For seniors, this is a golden opportunity to come back to normal life. Most seniors live a retired life and become depressed due to lack of activity. Exercise can provide them with a hobby and bring back excitement in their lives.

As a matter of fact, exercise is a common remedy against depression, distress, and emotional problems. During exercise, selected neurotransmitters are stimulated which lead to serenity.

Moreover, exercise can also induce relaxation in the body. This added relaxation can bring in a satiated sleep, which can greatly help seniors recover their lost energy levels. Exercise results in an increased amount of oxygen and blood being carried to the brain, which means the brain can now work more efficiently and without any stress.

# Chapter # 2: Comprehensive List

The following is the complete list of physical benefits induced by exercise:

- Prevents chronic diseases and other disabilities

- It helps bring down the risk of cardiovascular diseases

- It decreases the blood pressure

- It improves insulin and glucose metabolism which aids in bringing down the risk of diseases like diabetes

- It reduces the risk of osteoporosis by strengthening bones

- It brings back the physical power required to carry out day to day chores

- It increases balance which means a reduction in the risk of falling down

- It improves body composition

- It reduces the pain that comes with chronic pain syndromes

- It enhances immunity

Benefiting the body physically is not the only thing exercise is good at; here are a few psychological benefits that come with exercise:

- It decreases depression

- It enhances one's mood

- It increases cognitive ability

- It increases personal control in an individual

- It increases mental well-being

- Decreases stress

- It improves one's quality of life

- It adds to a person's sleep

# Chapter # 3: Falling Down

Falling down is a common phenomenon. Many times during exercises or in general, people fall down and instead of acting logically with calm, they tend to panic which causes emotional as well as physical harm. The person may not receive any injury from the fall itself, but might just get injured by the way he/she reacts after the fall. Therefore it is absolutely important that the person behave in a normal way if he/she falls down. Here is a set of information which will help you get back up to your feet, safely in case you fall:

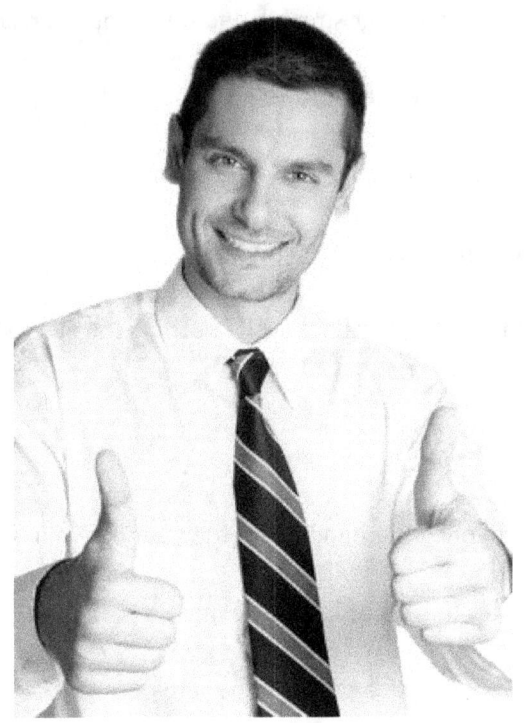

1.      Take a deep breath while laying still

2.      Try to relax

3. Start analyzing the situation and try to find out if you have gotten injured

4. If you have sustained an injury then do not attempt to get up but instead:

    i. Call emergency services

    ii. If you can't call someone to help you

    iii. If no one is around then lay there until you regain the strength to get up

5. When you regain your strength and think you are ready to get up:

    i. Roll over to either side by turning your head in either direction

    ii. Try to crawl to a chair, a sofa, or any solid object near you

    iii. Slowly pull your body upwards

    iv. Bend the stronger knee while keeping the other knee on the floor

    v. Slowly try to stand up

    vi. Twist yourself around and settle your body on the object

    vii. Now try to call for help once more

6. Make sure you visit a doctor to be sure of injuries.

# Aerobic Training

## Chapter # 1: Introduction

Aerobic exercise is a type of physical activity that engages large muscles of the body like the legs and shoulders to cause an increase in heart rate. The training is also known as endurance, cardiorespiratory, and cardiovascular training. This training is highlighted by simple activities like swimming, cycling, walking, climbing, etc. For elders, walking is the most recommended type of exercise since it does not require any special skills. This section will focus on walking exercises and advise you in ways through which the body can be maintained.

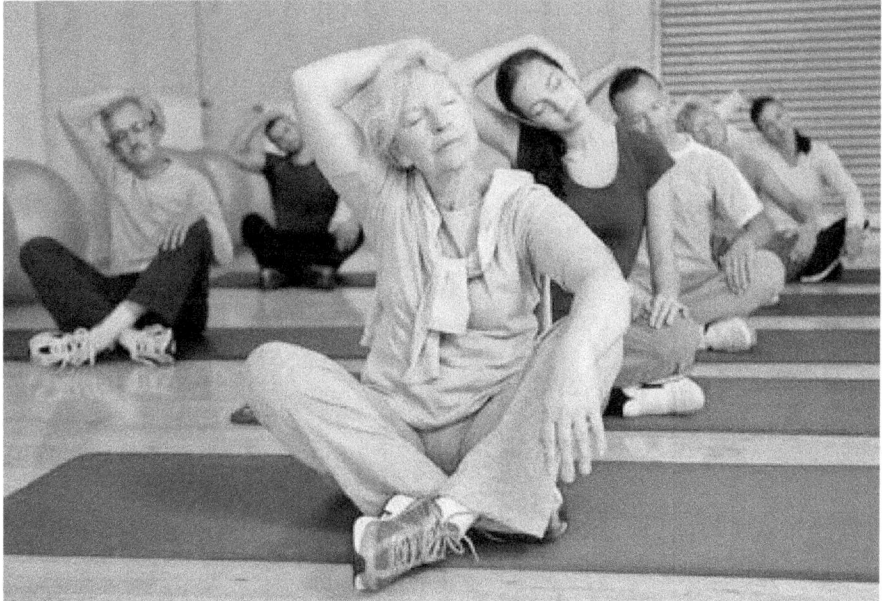

Walking is an excellent activity for elders and the biggest reason for this statement is the safety that's associated with it. It is an easy exercise and is basically something we're most experienced at. Right from childhood a person learns to walk and keeps walking his/her entire life. Walking can bring great medical benefits to the body like lowering the risk of heart disease, premature death, etc.

**Beginning to Walk:**

Walking as an exercise is very effective, but a few steps should be kept in mind before engaging in this physical activity:

1. Walk short distances, at first: When starting walking as a physical activity, start slow and gradually increase your distance as time progresses.

2. Walk at nominal pace: Don't compromise quality over quantity, so focus on your posture and walk at a comfortable pace.

3. Talk during walking: Always try to talk during walks and if you find difficulty in doing so then you are walking way too fast.

# Chapter # 2: Weeks 1, 2 & 3

**Week 1:**

You do not need to walk for 30 minutes at a time to get the benefits associated with walking. You are allowed to break up the walking time into smaller units and spread them throughout the day. For instance, you may walk 10 minutes during the morning, 10 after lunch and 10 before dinner; it's up to you. Here are a few things that should be kept in mind during the first week:

1.  Your goal throughout the regimen should be to record your steps. Every morning reset the pedometer to ZERO and set it to record your steps; ignore other settings. Close the pedometer and attach it to your waist to the right or the left of the kneecap. Wear it all day long and as night approaches, record the steps.

2.  The first week should be composed of the normal routine, do not rush into anything and be calm. Record the steps each day and remember to have your pedometer with you each day.

3.  During the weekend, the natural desire of the body is to rest but you must be able to fight this desire if the step numbers on the pedometer are low.

**Week 2:**

The goal you have to achieve every 1 – 2 weeks is a 10 percent increase in the average number of steps. The new target should be set by keeping in mind the average number of steps a day in the previous week. For instance, if you clock 800 steps a day in week A, then you should aim for 880 steps a day in the subsequent week. Here are few things to have in mind during the second week:

1. Start increasing your steps by employing tactics like parking the car further, playing with a pet, etc. Have your pedometer assist with the statistics.

2. Be more active; start volunteering in communities and other activities through which maximum steps can be obtained.

3. Also try to engage in other aerobic activities if the body allows you. For instance, you may start to take yoga classes, dancing lessons or any other activity that increases physical exposure.

**Week 3:**

Your final goal after a number of weeks should be 10,000 steps a day! That's a huge goal, but at the pace stated in Week 2, it would take 6 months to 1 year. If the secondary goal of your workout is weight loss then you'll have to increase your steps by 10 percent; otherwise if the goal is aerobic fitness then you'll have to increase your walking speed. Here are a few tips for week 3:

1. The 10,000 steps a day should be your benchmark for better health. The general instruction for you is to keep on increasing steps by 10 percent. But, there are plenty of chance that you'll break the 10,000 steps barrier, so if you want to, you may aim for higher ground.

2. In order to keep increasing the number of steps, you'll have to make good lifestyle choices as well. For many people, a trip to a new

place can act as a catalyst in walking. For some, taking breaks can be beneficial; you'll have to find your own strong suit.

3.    Some days however, you might not feel like walking at all, and you should not panic upon feeling these emotions as this will be a part of your regiment. These days will come and go so keep yourself flexible. Instead of holding to a certain number of steps each day, allow the steps to fluctuate so that you're able to fill the void left by a low-stepping day. Remember, increasing the weekly average to 9000 steps from 8000 baseline steps is a great improvement.

# Chapter # 3: Sample Activity Log

Many people complain of not getting proper guidance, so here is a sample log which illustrates a 6 week schedule for walking. You may build one for yourself to keep track of your walking routine:

|  | *One* | *Two* | *Three* | *Four* | *Five* | *Six* |
|---|---|---|---|---|---|---|
| *Monday* | 10 minutes | 15 minutes | 20 minutes | 20 minutes | 25 minutes | 20 minutes |
| *Tuesday* | 10 minutes | 15 minutes | 20 minutes | 20 minutes | Rest | 30 minutes |
| *Wednesday* | 10 minutes | Rest | Rest | 20 minutes | 25 minutes | 30 minutes |
| *Thursday* | Rest | 20 minutes | 20 minutes | Rest | 25 minutes | 30 minutes |
| *Friday* | 15 minutes | 20 minutes | 15 minutes | Rest | 25 minutes | 10 minutes |
| *Saturday* | Rest | Rest | 20 minutes | 25 minutes | 25 minutes | Rest |
| *Sunday* | 15 minutes | 20 minutes | 20 minutes | 25 minutes | Rest | 30 minutes |
| *TOTALS* | 60 minutes | 90 minutes | 115 minutes | 110 minutes | 150 minutes | 150 minutes |

# Strength Training

## Chapter # 1: Introduction

Strength training is defined as a type of physical activity which involves the person using resistance to build strength in the body. The strength is complimented by the size of skeletal muscles and anaerobic endurance. This section introduces another type of exercise and is designed in a manner which will allow you to engage in home based training. But, before diving right into the program, a few safety considerations must be looked over.

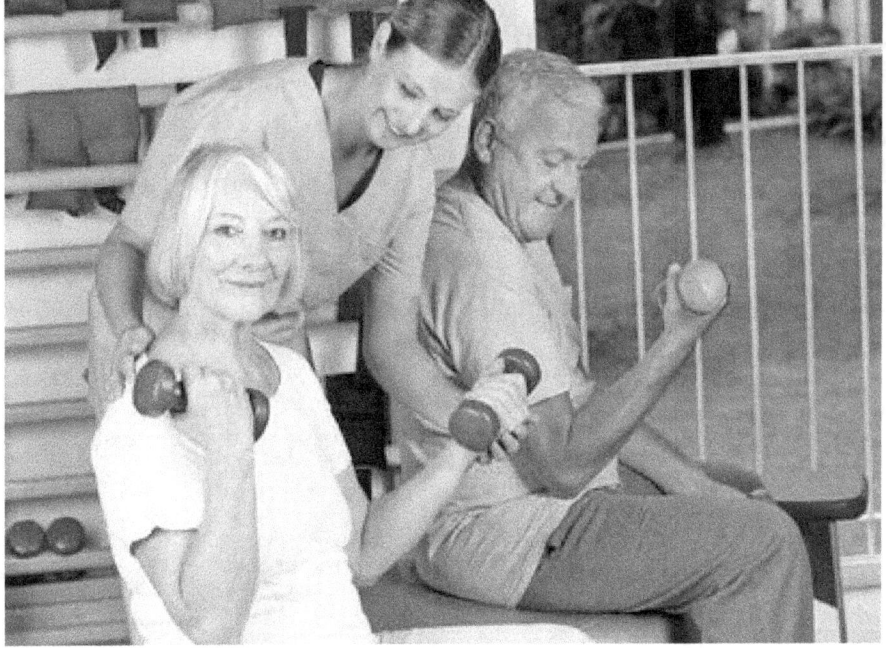

1. Before starting the regimen, visit a doctor and get clearance from him/her first, regarding the nature of the exercise.

2. Stop exercising if you notice the following signs:

i.     Dizziness

ii.    Numbness

iii.   Chest pains

iv.    Joint pains

v.     Heart racing at an irregular speed

The training program is to be carried out 2 to 3 times in a week. It should take 20 to 30 minutes or longer depending on the time you take to warm up as well as rest in-between sets. Each exercise would be performed for 8 – 15 reps. If a weight is too heavy and you are unable to execute 8 reps then try lifting a lighter weight. If 15 reps are performed for each exercise then choose a heavier weight. After completing 8 – 15 reps, rest for 1 – 2 minutes before repeating the reps again. Each 8 reps are known as sets and the book recommends 1 – 2 sets for each exercise you perform.

There are also a few general conditions you should have in your mind before initiating strength training exercises using weights:

i.     When sitting, a little portion of the back should be pressed firmly against the chair back

ii.    When standing, the natural arch in the back should be maintained

iii.   When lying, a little portion of the back should be pressed up firmly against the surface of the floor

iv.    Each movement should be carried out with complete concentration and control

v.      Resist gravity and don't allow a weight to fall freely

vi.     Spend about 3 seconds when lifting a weight and almost the same amount when dropping it

vii.    Breathe during lifting

viii.   Don't hold your breathe.

Your warm up should consist of walking, marching, or cycling at a low pace which would be necessary to get the muscles warm. The next sections explain the exercises that need to be carried out. If you have concerns about any of the exercises, it is best you see a medical expert. Pick two exercises at the start and slowly build up your endurance to carry them all out.

The following are the Upper body exercises explained in the book:

-       Seated lateral rise

-       Biceps curl

-       One arm triceps

-       Shoulder shrugs

-       Chest press

-       One arm row

-       Abdominal crunch

The following are the Lower body exercises explained in the book:

-       Heel raises

- Leg extensions

- Hamstring curls

- Body weight squats

- Gluteal extension

# Chapter # 2: Upper Body Exercises

First off are the upper body exercises which focus on providing extra strength to the upper portion of the body like the chest, shoulders, and arms.

**1.    Seated Lateral Raise:**

This exercise is for the shoulders and here are the steps to it:

i.    Pick a chair without arm rests and sit on it. Make sure that a small portion of the back is in contact with the back of the chair. The body should be aligned straight with the shoulders resting back. Your main focus should be in the forward direction with the chin up and away from the chest. The feet should be placed flat on the ground and shoulder-width apart.

ii.    Have the weights in each hand and arms by your side; form a perpendicular angle between the upper arm and the forearm and get ready to execute.

iii.    Take a deep breath and slowly exhale as you raise the weight keeping your arms straight out to the side; hold at the top for a second.

iv.    Now slowly return it to the starting point while inhaling.

**2.    Biceps curl:**

This exercise is for the upper arms and targets the front portion.

i.    Once again, pick a chair without arm rests and sit down. Also be sure to have a small portion of the back in contact with the chair. Focus upfront, and have your chest aligned.

ii.     Have weights in both hands and position your arms straight by your side, keeping the elbows pressed up against the side of your body.

iii.    Take a deep breath and raise your forearms while exhaling; hold at this position for 1 second.

iv.     Once again, return to the starting position.

**3.     Shoulder shrugs:**

This exercise is aimed or the upper back as well as the shoulders:

i.      Pick a seat that does not have arm rests; press a small portion of the back to the chair and keep your body straight. Have your focus right in front of you and place your feet on the floor, shoulder width apart.

ii.     Have weights in both hands, arms by the side and take a deep breathe.

iii.    Maintain a nominal distance between the chest and the chin and slowly shrug the shoulders; exhale.

iv.     Imagine as if you were about to lift the shoulders to your ears without altering the head position at all; slowly lower your shoulders to the starting position and inhale.

**4.     One arm triceps:**

This exercise is aimed for the back of the upper arms and is executed as follows:

i.      Take a seat in a chair that doesn't have any arm rests. Press a small portion of the back against the chair, have your chest aligned and focus in the forward direction. Feet should be shoulder width apart.

ii.     This time, pick up only one weight and hold the arm directly over your shoulder, with the elbow pointing in a 60 degree angle towards the ceiling; the opposite arm should support this elbow.

iii.    Straighten the arm with the weight slowly while exhaling.

iv.     Take a deep breath and lower the arm to the starting point.

**5.     One Arm Row:**

This exercise is designed for the back and the shoulders:

i.      Stand next to a solid object like a table or a sofa and with the feet shoulder width apart, place your hand on the surface and bend your waist perpendicularly. Keep your shoulders as well as head up and maintain a nominal space between the chest and the chin.

ii.     Extend the free arm forward and hold the weight in this hand.

iii.    Take a deep breathe, exhale, and slowly start to draw your elbows which would straighten the back.

iv.     Hold in this position for a second before slowly returning to the starting position; remember to inhale as you return.

**6.     Chest press:**

As the name suggests, this exercise is designed for the chest:

i.    Lie down on your bed while facing up; place your feet flat on the surface and bend your knees until the back is firmly in contact with the bed.

ii.   Focus forward and keep your chin away from your chest.

iii.  Hold weights in your hands and bring your arms to the side making a 90 degree angle between the forearms as well as upper arms.

iv.   Take a deep breathe, exhale as you press your arms forward; keep pressing until the side of the weights come together above your chest.

v.    Inhale and start to return to the initial point where you started.

# Chapter # 3: Lower Body Exercises

Now for the lower body activities which would be to strengthen the lower body muscles, joints, etc. Here are the exercises:

1. **Leg extension:**

This exercise focusses on the upper front part of the legs:

i.  Pick a chair that doesn't have any arm rests. Be sure to have a small part of your back in contact with the chair. The body should be kept straight and the shoulders should be aligned sideways. Your focus should always be in the forward direction away from the chest. Lastly, both the feet should be flat on the floor.

ii.  You should have your ankle weights secured to each ankle.

iii.  Hold the chair with both hands but don't grip it too tightly.

iv.  Take a deep breath and while exhaling slowly straighten one of the legs. Maintain distance between the knees and do not let them touch.

v.  Hold the horizontal position for a few seconds before coming back to the starting position.

vi.  The number of repetitions to be executed is up to you.

2. **Heel raises:**

This exercise is designed for the calves or the bottom back of the legs; here are the steps:

i. Find a secure surface like a table or a sofa and stand next to it. Keep the feet at least shoulder width apart and the body perfectly straight. Now put on the ankle weights and place your hands on a secure surface and keep your head erect.

ii. Take a deep breath and slowly start to raise your heels off the surface of the ground whilst taking the chair's support; keep lifting yourself until you stand on your toes.

iii. Maintain a stable posture throughout the movement.

iv. Hold the position for a second before returning to the starting position; remember to inhale as you return.

## 3. Hamstrings Curls:

This exercise is for the upper back of the legs:

i. Find a stable surface and stand next to it with feet shoulders width apart. With the ankle weights on, place each hand on a secure surface while keeping your head erect.

ii. Take a deep breath and raise your heel off the ground until the angle between the upper and lower body is 90 degree.

iii. Exhale through the movement.

iv. Hold this position for a second or two before returning to the original one.

v. Do as many reps as you want.

## 4. Body weight squat:

This exercise is aimed for the legs and the bottom part; it is as follows:

i.      Pick a chair whose seat is located just above your knee; stand with the feet shoulder width apart with the heels 5 inches in front of the chair. Stand straight with the shoulders aligned sideways and focus in the forward direction.

ii.      Inhale as slowly as you can and start to bend your knees; slowly sit on the chair, maintaining control while lowering. Extend the arms forward so that they act like counter balances.

iii.      Stop the movement when the back of your legs are in contact with the chair. Sometimes for starters, it is not possible to bring the body back up so it's okay to rest a little.

iv.      When returning, exhale.

**5.     Gluteal Extension:**

This exercise is aimed for the legs and the bottom part; it is as follows:

i.      Find a secure surface and stand next to it; keep the feet shoulder width apart and stand straight. With the ankles weights on, place your hands on the surface and keep your head erect.

ii.      Now, take a breath and extend the nearer leg backwards as far as you can without bending your waist. Maintain an erect posture throughout the movement.

iii.      Hold for one second at the position before returning to the initial point.

iv.      After a certain number of reps, switch the legs.

## 6.     Abdominal crunch:

This exercise, as the name suggests, is for the abdominal muscles:

i.      Lie on your bed facing upwards and place the sole of the feet on the surface of the bed; adjust the angle until your back is firmly in contact with the bed. Be sure to have concentration in the forward direction.

ii.     Your hands should be placed behind your skull and while breathing, lift your torso off the bed so that you squeeze your abdominal muscles.

iii.    Try to imagine a string pulling you upwards from your chest towards the ceiling of the room.

iv.     Hold onto this position for a few seconds before inhaling and coming back to the original position.

# Conclusion

Aging is a natural phenomenon that all of us have to face at some point in our lives. With aging comes a host of conditions which signal that the body is no longer as energetic, young, and jubilant as it once used to be. A person needs to accept this fact and if he swallows this hard truth he/she can see that there's light beyond this tunnel of fragility. This book explains just that. The book starts off by telling the basic advantages of physical activity. If a normal aged person can reap all these benefits then imagine what an older structure can get. Subsequently, the book tells about the two major types of physical activities that an elderly person can engage in to attain better fitness. The exercises explained belong either to the aerobic type or the strength type, but both of them will help you regain lost stamina and power. You just need to put in the time and you'll start to feel like you're having a new beginning. To achieve that you'll have to motivate yourself to get up from your bed or couch and just do it.

Best of luck, stay healthy!

# Author Bio

Muhammad Usman is a distinguished medical graduate of Allama Iqbal medical college (AIMC). He is a professional writer who has been in the field for more than 4 years. During this time he has produced 10,000+ articles, blogs and eBooks on various niches related to diseases, health, fitness, nutrition and well-being. He is a regular contributor to several journals related to medicine and surgery. He is the editor of several journals and newspapers.

# References

1. http://www.fotolia.com/id/39676947

2. http://www.fotolia.com/id/49218655

3. http://www.fotolia.com/id/51102457

4. http://www.fotolia.com/id/45257208

5. http://www.fotolia.com/id/39332640

6. http://www.fotolia.com/id/46908327

Check out some of the other JD-Biz Publishing books

Gardening Series on Amazon

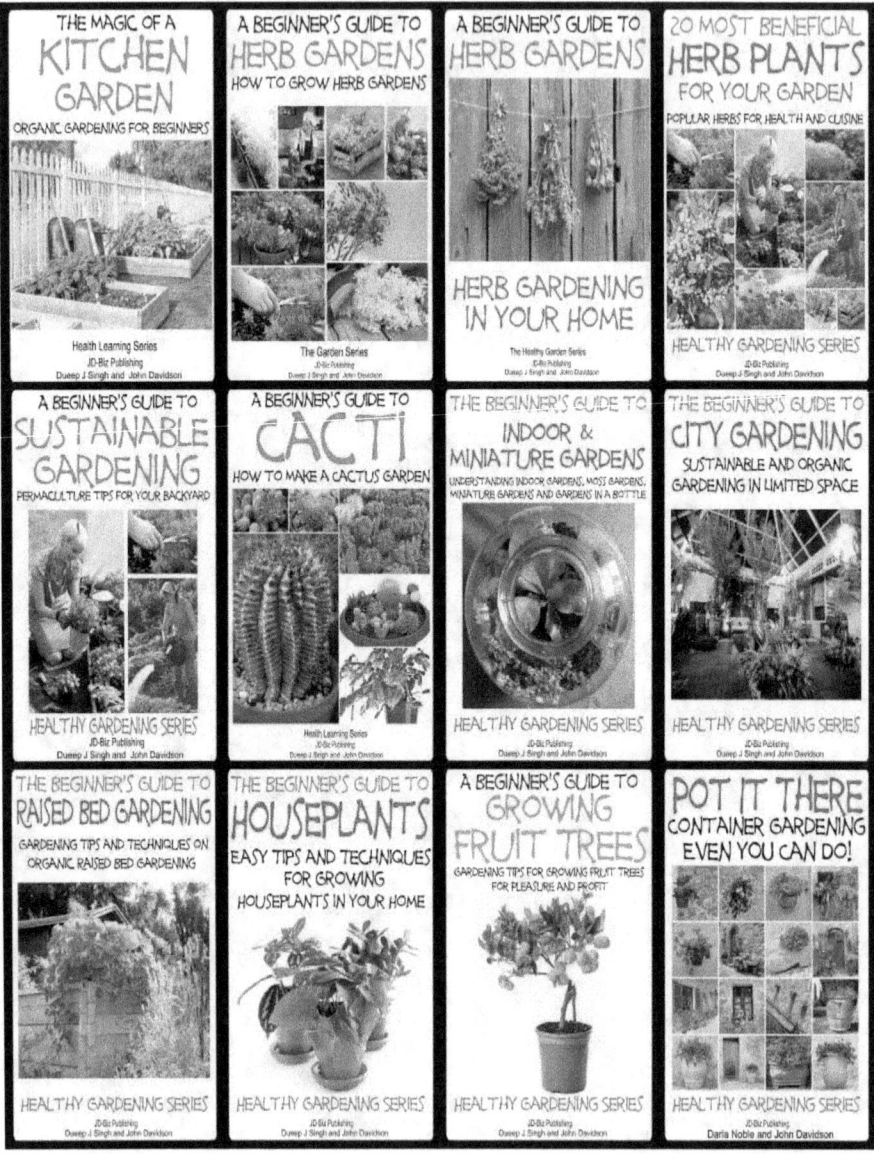

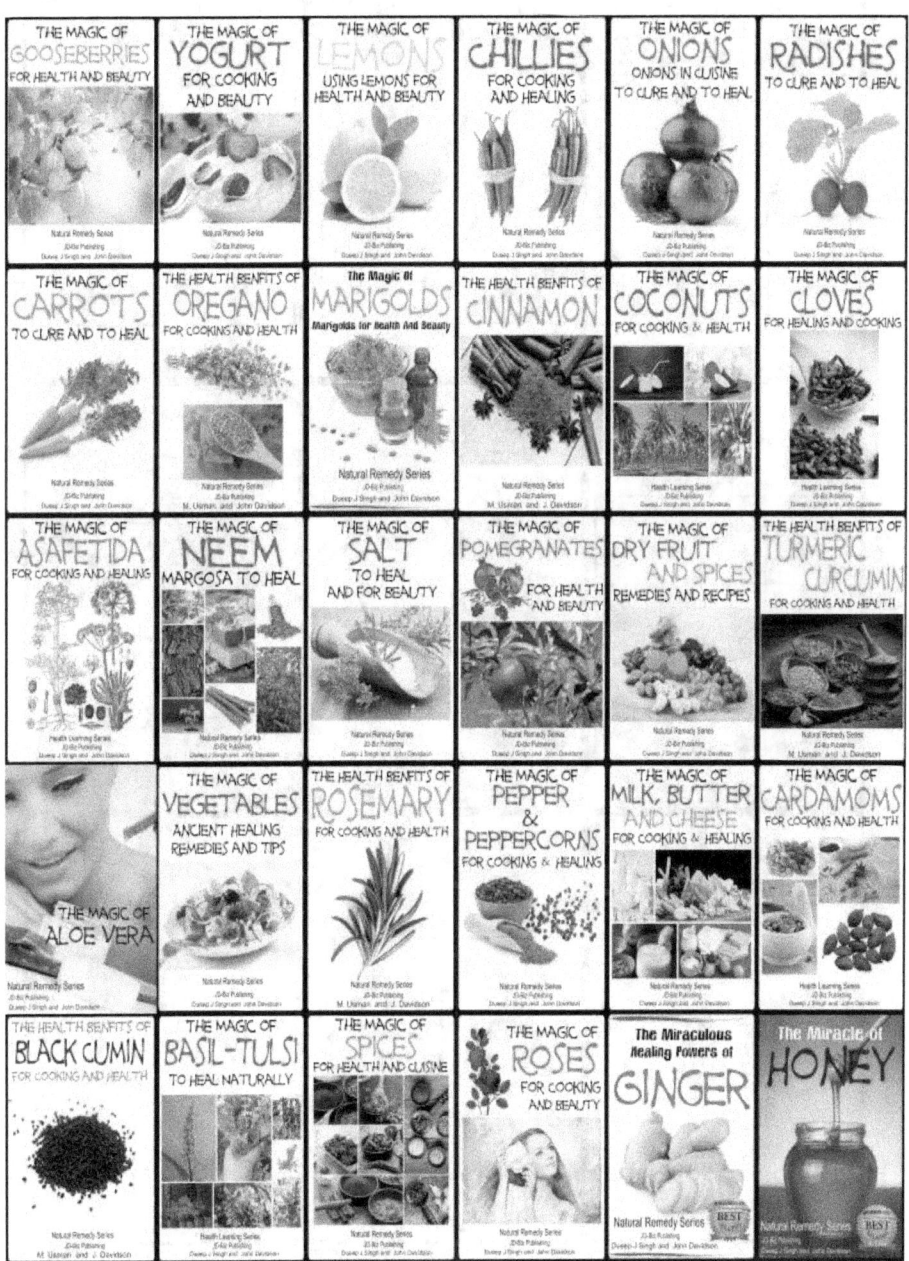

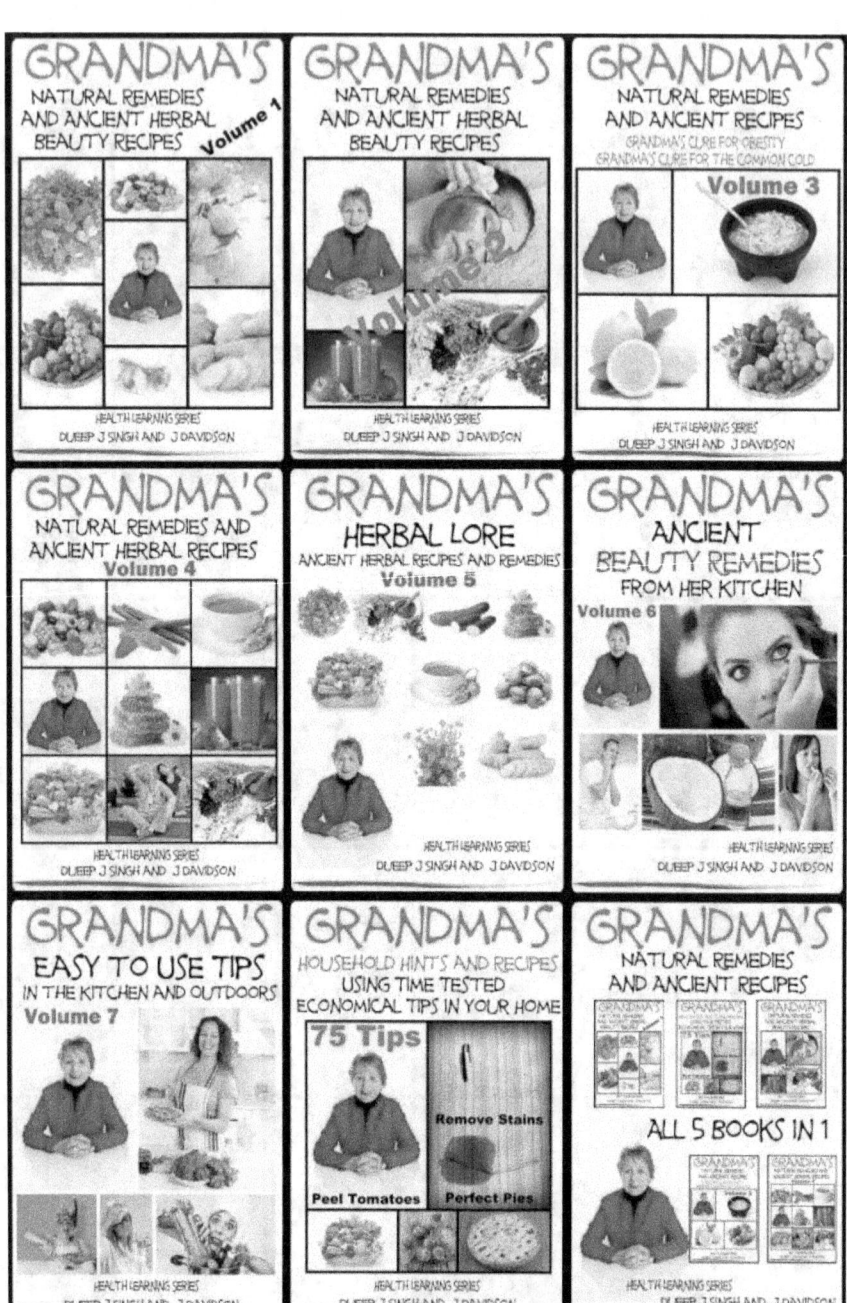

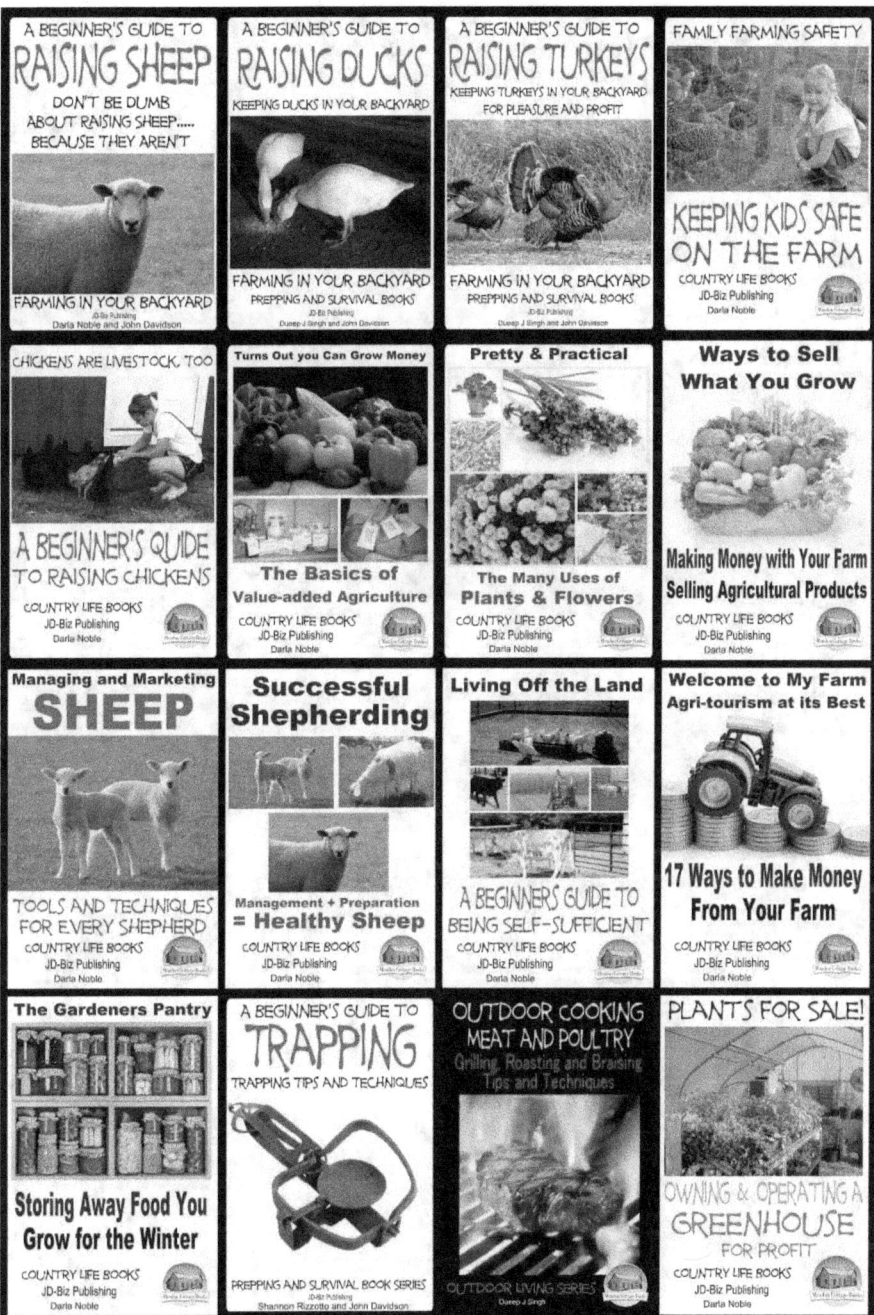

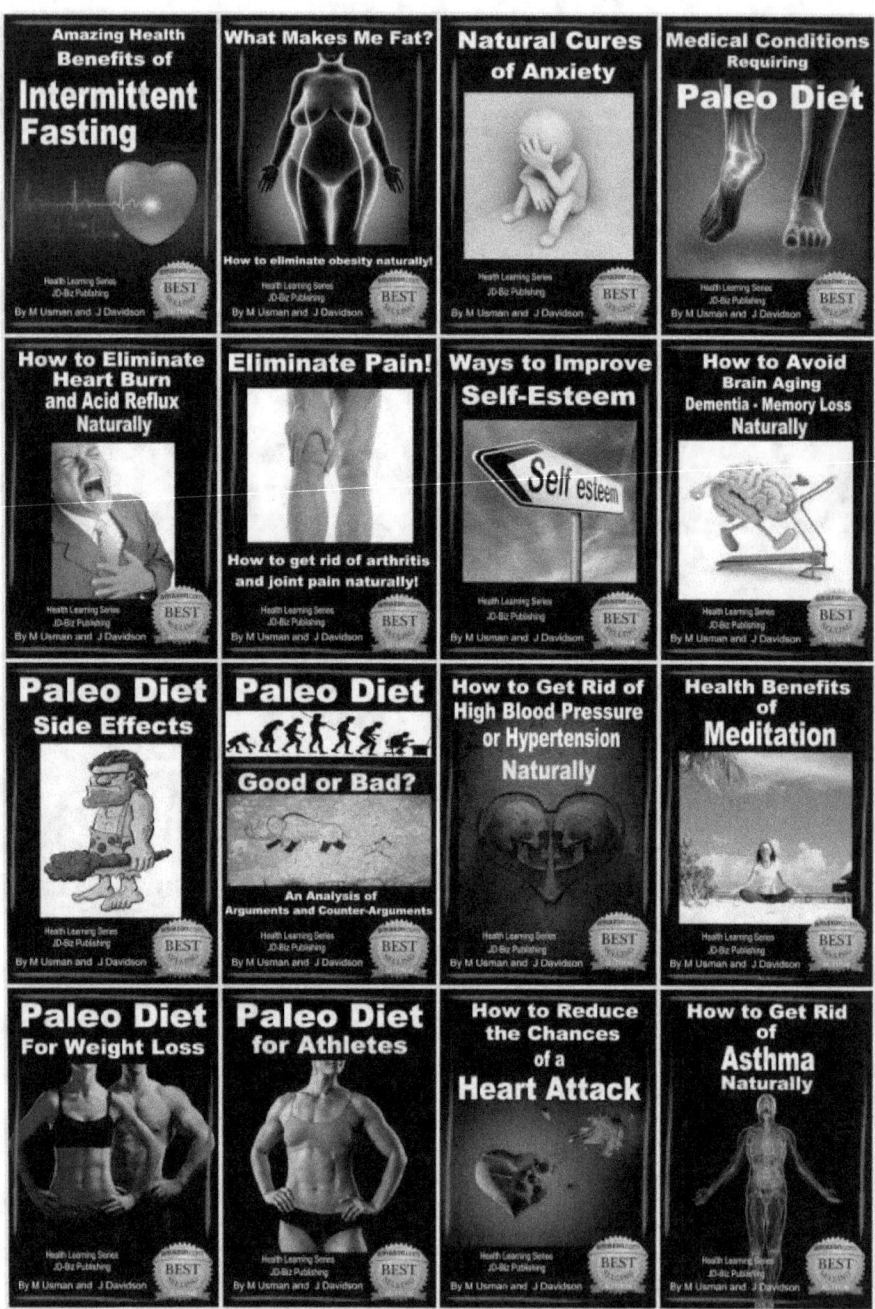

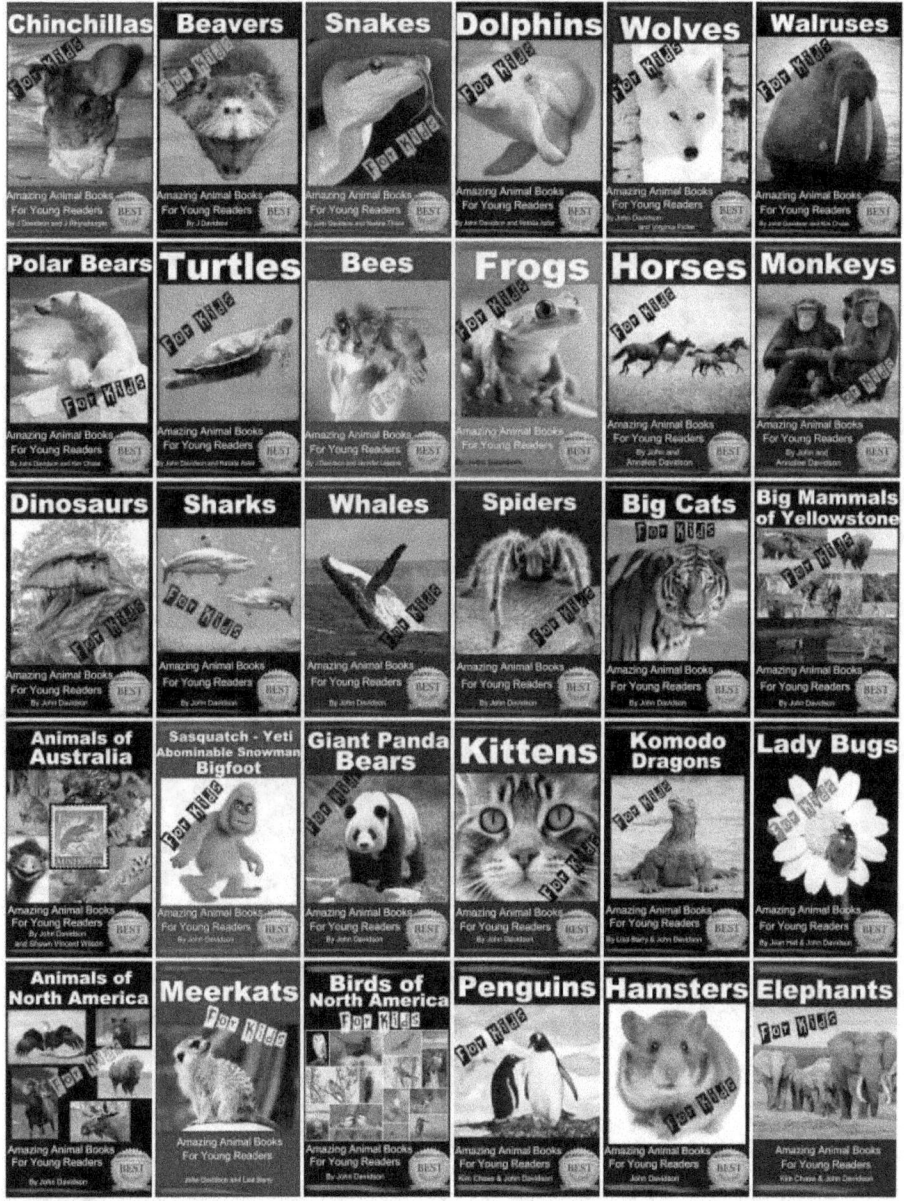

# Learn To Draw Series

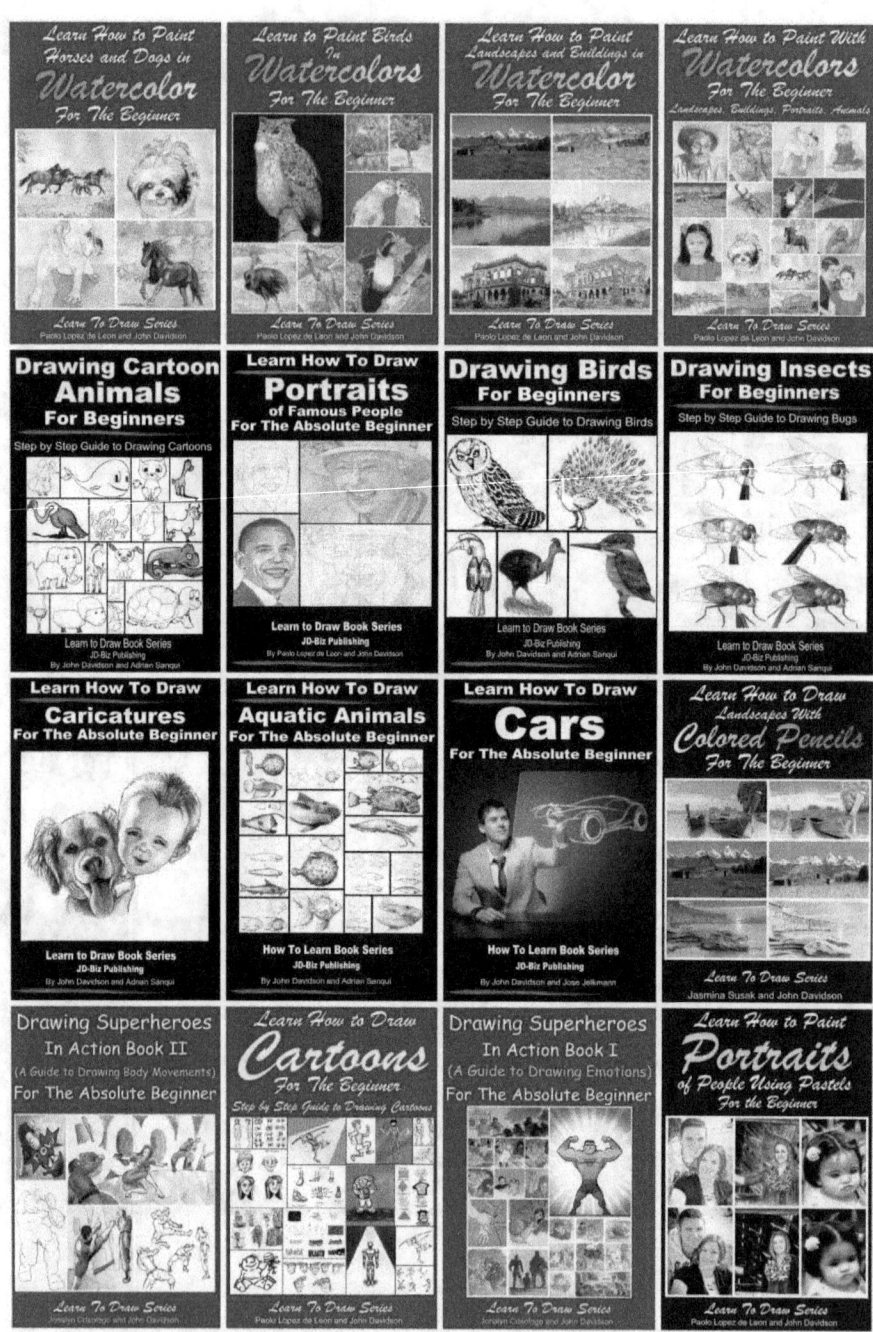

# How to Build and Plan Books

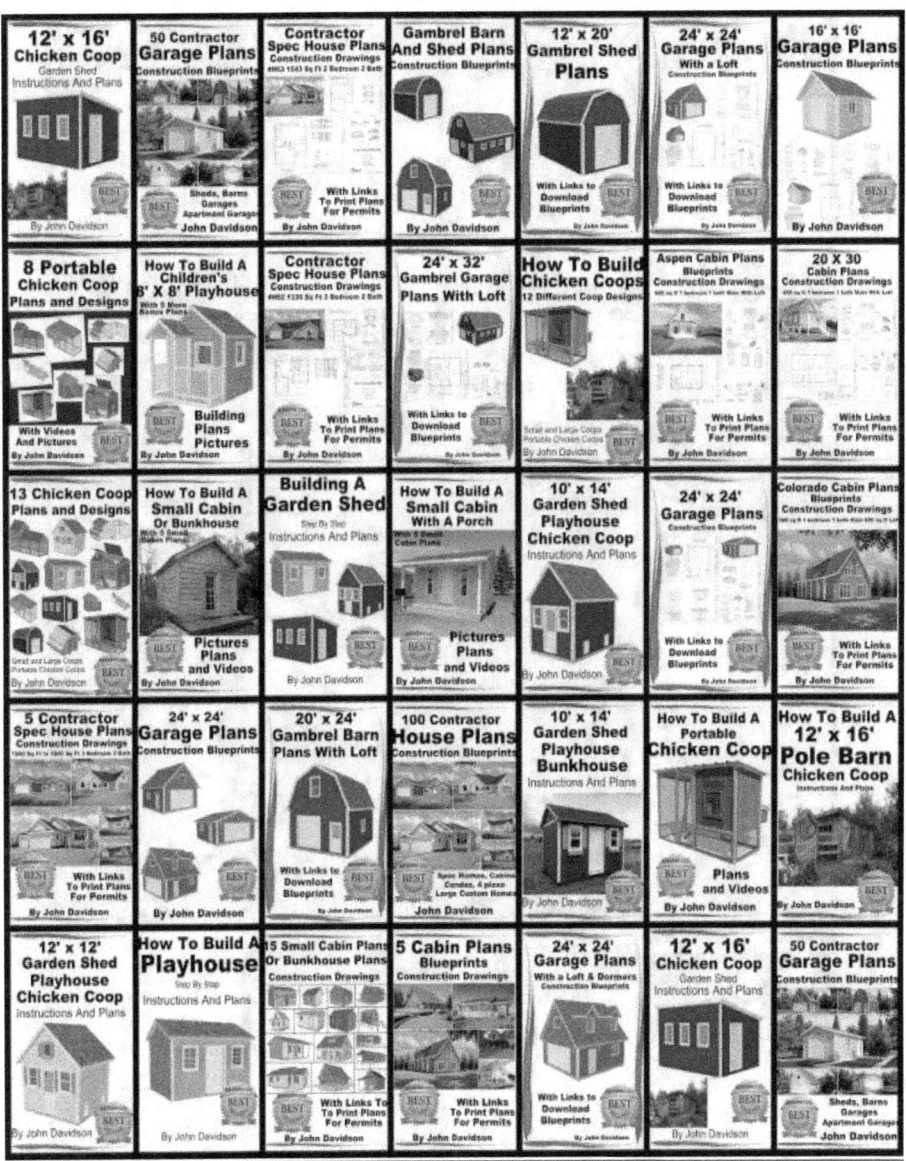

# Entrepreneur Book Series

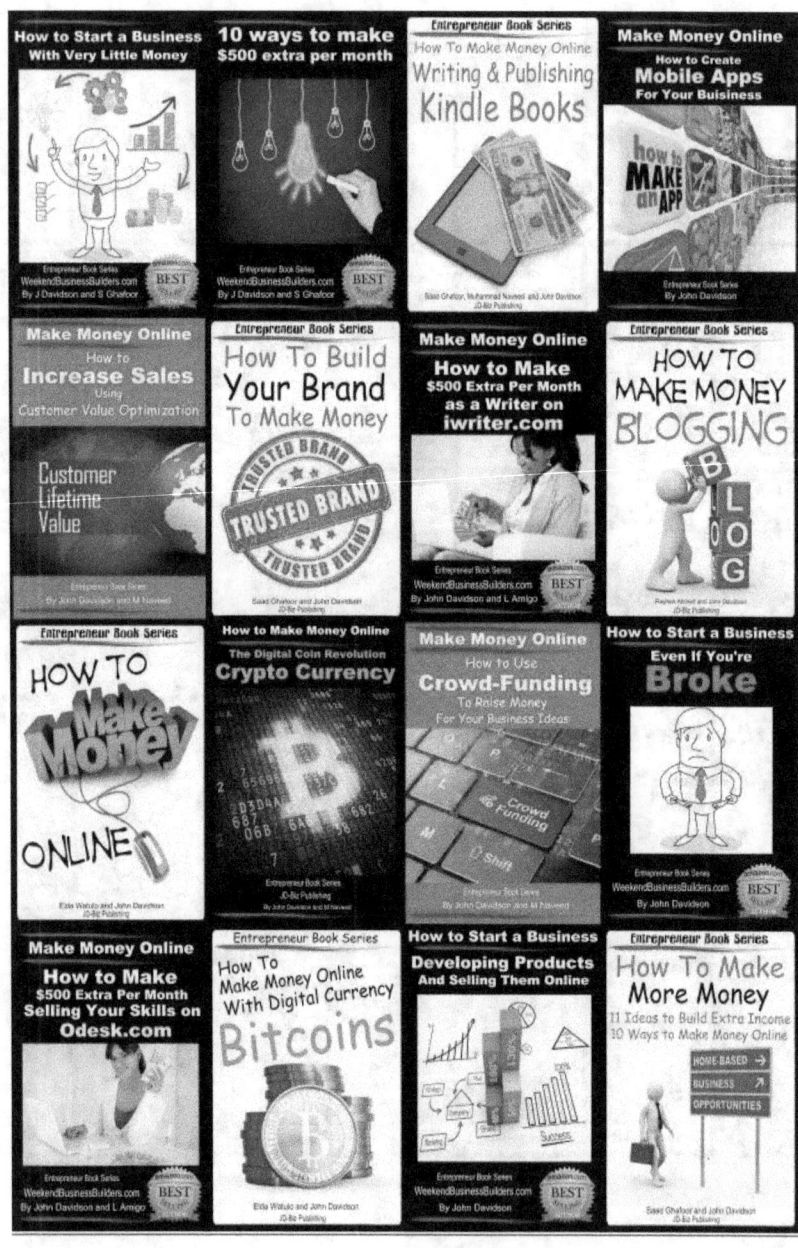

Our books are available at

1. Amazon.com

2. Barnes and Noble

3. Itunes

4. Kobo

5. Smashwords

6. Google Play Books

# Publisher

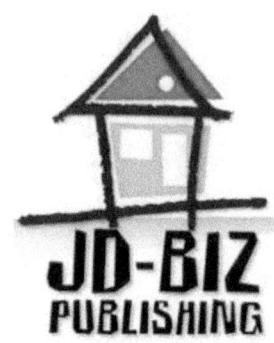

JD-Biz Corp

P O Box 374

Mendon, Utah 84325

http://www.jd-biz.com/

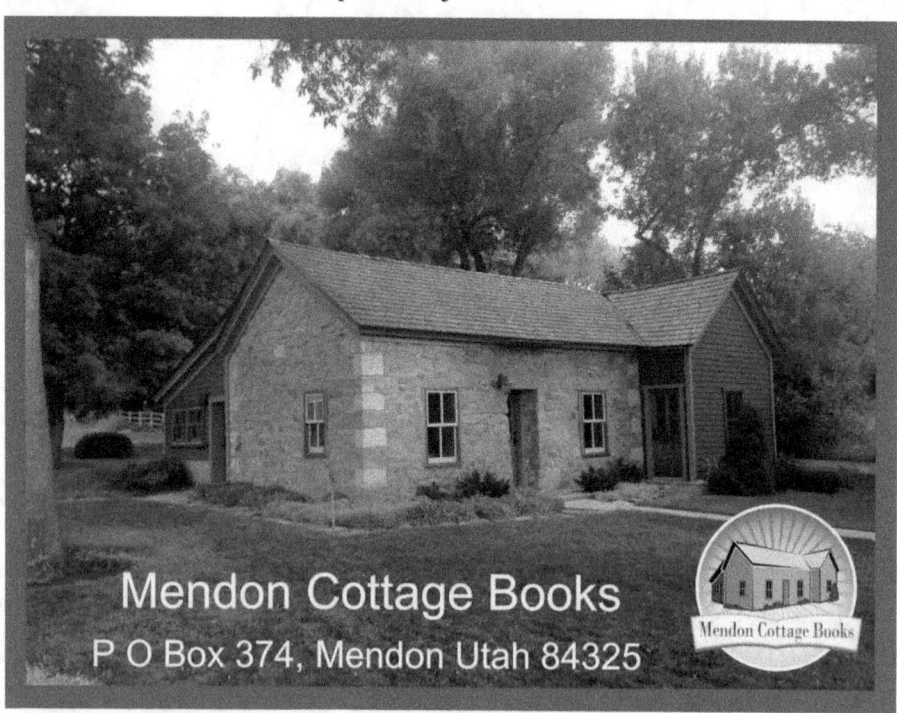

Mendon Cottage Books

P O Box 374, Mendon Utah 84325

www.ingramcontent.com/pod-product-compliance
Lightning Source LLC
Chambersburg PA
CBHW072251310526
45795CB00011B/940